Lata Kumari
Shalini Garg
Vishal Sharma

Eruption Disturbances Of Teeth In Children

Lata Kumari
Shalini Garg
Vishal Sharma

Eruption Disturbances Of Teeth In Children

A Guide To Disturbances In Tooth Eruption In Children.

LAP LAMBERT Academic Publishing

Cover image: www.ingimage.com

Publisher:
LAP LAMBERT Academic Publishing
is a trademark of
Dodo Books Indian Ocean Ltd. and OmniScriptum S.R.L publishing group

120 High Road, East Finchley, London, N2 9ED, United Kingdom
Str. Armeneasca 28/1, office 1, Chisinau MD-2012, Republic of Moldova, Europe
Managing Directors: Ieva Konstantinova, Victoria Ursu
info@omniscriptum.com

Printed at: see last page
ISBN: 978-620-8-44075-6

ACKNOWLEDGEMENT

Writing this library dissertation has been fascinating and extremely rewarding. I would like to thank a number of people who have contributed to the final result in many different ways.

I would like to express my deepest gratitude to all those who have contributed to the completion of this dissertation.

First and foremost, I would like to extend my heartfelt thanks to my guide **Dr. Shalini Garg** for her invaluable support, guidance and encouragement throughout this research. Her expertise, constructive criticism, and constant motivation helped me shape this dissertation and push my academic boundaries.

I am also grateful to my co-guide **Dr. Vishal Sharma**, whose insightful feedback and suggestions were instrumental in enhancing the quality of my work. His guidance helped me maintain focus and direction in my research.

A sincere thanks goes to the Head of the Department **Dr. Anil Gupta** for providing the necessary resources and a conducive environment for my research. His leadership and vision have been a source of inspiration during my academic journey.

My deepest gratitude to my parents **Mr. Jaibir Singh** and **Mrs. Usha** and my sister **Bhawna** and brother **Vipin** for their unflagging love and unconditional support throughout the journey so that I could study and focus on my work.
I would like to express my sincere gratitude to my senior **Dr. Prince Rathee** for his invaluable guidance and support throughout the course of my dissertation. His advice, encouragement, and willingness to share his knowledge and resources from the library greatly contributed to the success of this work.

I am truly grateful for the time and effort he dedicated in helping me understand complex concepts, providing useful references, and guiding me in the right direction whenever I faced challenges. Thank you once again for being a constant source of support and inspiration during this academic journey.

I would like to express my heartfelt gratitude to my friend and batchmate **Dr. Shweta** for her constant support, encouragement, and valuable suggestions throughout this dissertation. Her help and motivation made this journey smoother and more memorable. And also, thanks go to my batchmates **Dr. Anshula, Dr Mahima, Dr. Minakshi and Dr. Nidhi.**

I would also like to acknowledge the support and cooperation of my seniors **Dr. Neha, Dr. Mansi, Dr. Sakshi Jainer, Dr. Sakshi Singla, Dr. Anushi** and lovely juniors **Dr. Vibhusha, Dr. Nikita, Dr. Jyoti, Dr. Savari, Dr. Medha and Dr. Muskan** for their timely assistance in clinics and otherwise. Their patience and willingness to help made a significant difference in the completion of this dissertation.

Also, my thanks go to assistants of our department **Mr. Manish, Mr. Darshan, Mr. Manveer and Mr. Vikas**.

Above all, I owe it all to Almighty God for granting me the wisdom, health and strength to undertake this research task and enabling me for its completion. I am truly grateful to everyone who played a part in this endeavour.

Dr. Lata kumari

. List of Contributors

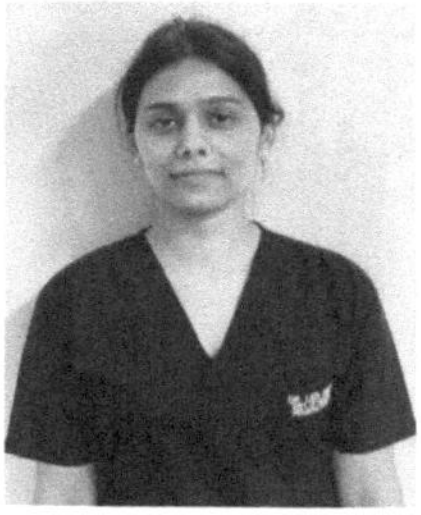

Dr. Lata Kumari
Post Graduate Student
Department of Pediatric & Preventive Dentistry
Faculty of Dental Sciences, SGT University,
Gurugram, Haryana, India

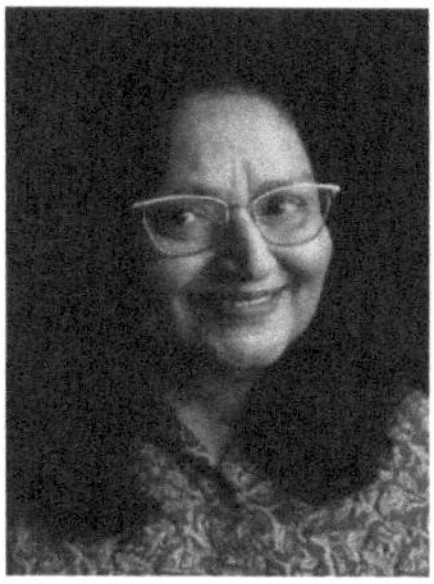

Dr. Shalini Garg
Professor
Department of Pediatric & Preventive Dentistry
Faculty of Dental Sciences, SGT University,
Gurugram, Haryana, India

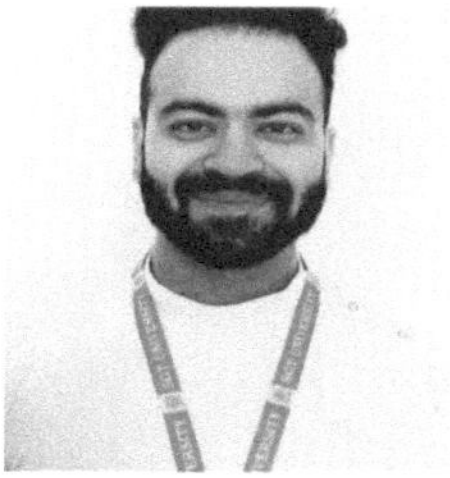

Dr. Vishal Sharma
Senior Lecturer
Department of Pediatric & Preventive Dentistry
Faculty of Dental Sciences, SGT University,
Gurugram, Haryana, India

CONTENTS

LEGENDS
LIST OF FIGURES

INTRODUCTION

The physiological process known as dental eruption occurs when a tooth is vertically moved from its initial non-functional, developing position to its functional position to occlude with its antagonist.[1] The phrase "tooth eruption" is frequently used to describe a condition, when a tooth first appears in the oral cavity. This displacement occurs through the oral epithelium and the alveolar process. [2] A series of communication events between the osteoblast and the osteoclast cells of the alveolar process occur in synchrony during the tooth eruption process.[3]

A child's development is said to reach a significant milestone when the deciduous teeth erupt, exfoliate and is followed by the eruption of the permanent dentition. This process is sequential and age-specific.[4] Primary teeth usually erupt at about six months of age. Premature eruption of primary teeth (dentitio praecox) has no significant cause behind it. It is most likely the result of numerous local and universal variables. [5,6]

Premature eruption is most commonly explained by the superficial position of the tooth germ, which is most likely inherited. The effects of congenital syphilis, endocrine disorders, dietary inadequacies, hypovitaminosis and a higher rate of eruption during or following feverish episodes can all be linked to the early eruption of primary teeth. It is also thought to be caused by environmental pollutants, particularly dibenzofurans & polychlorinated biphenyls. [7]

Either primary retention or secondary retention can be used to describe tooth eruption failure.[8] When a tooth fails to erupt locally without the concurrence of any other local or systemic reason, this is known as initial eruption discontinuation. Initial eruption failure of the teeth has been linked to idiopathic eruption failure.[9]

In some newborns, teeth that are present at birth are termed as natal teeth, whereas in some they erupt 30 days postpartum and are termed as neonatal teeth.[9] Early infancy teeth, also known as precociously erupted primary teeth (dentition praecox), are teeth that erupt between one to three months after life. The existence of teeth in a neonate's oral cavity has also been referred to by a number of names, including preterm teeth, predeciduous teeth, fetal teeth, and congenital teeth. [10] Primary teeth make up around 90% of teeth that erupt prematurely, while supernumerary teeth make up 10%. With a ratio of roughly 3:1, natal teeth are more common than neonatal teeth. [11]

Genetic factors are frequently blamed for eruptive failure. Cleidocranial dysplasia, Gardner syndrome, osteoglophonic dwarfism, regional odontodysplasia, oculodental syndrome, Rutherfurd type, Nance–Horan syndrome, Cherubism, Albers-Schönberg osteopetrosis, McCune–Albright syndrome, hypodontia–dysplasia of nails syndrome, osteopetrosis, mucopolysaccharidosis, and GAPO syndrome are just a few of the numerous syndromes that have been identified to be involved in eruption failure. [12]

While there have been instances of early eruption, delayed tooth eruption is the most common deviation from the normal eruption time. The teeth must erupt in a timely and sequential fashion for the infant to grow generally. Variations can have numerous causes, but eruption delays more than two years should be investigated. Early childhood malnutrition and inadequate nutrition have an impact on tooth eruption and cause the teeth to erupt later than expected.[12]

A previously conducted study found about the genetic origin of primary failure of eruption, a rare condition characterized by partial tooth eruption despite the presence of a distinct eruption pathway. The major failure of eruption was linked to 51 distinct variants of the PTH1R (parathyroid hormone 1 receptor) gene.[13]

Significant tooth eruption delays brought on by systemic, local, and hereditary factors are the hallmark of delayed tooth emergence (DTE). DTE raises the risk of crowding and malocclusion, which can lead to a number of orthodontic as well as psychological effects on the patient, particularly if anterior teeth are impacted. For orthodontic treatment, a deeper comprehension of the etiology of DTE is essential. In fact, SNPs in the genes ADK, BMP4, MMP8, and RANKL were connected to DTE. Thus, there are reasonable theories that suggest SNPs in genes related to craniofacial development, including VDR, PTH, ESR1, and ESR2, may also be involved in DTE. [15]

The clinical practice may be impacted by the hunt for DTE biomarkers, which would help pediatric dentists to create individualized treatment plans for every child.

Chapter-1

PREMATURE ERUPTION

The physiological process of a tooth moving from its crypt during odontogenesis via the alveolar process to its functional position in the oral cavity is commonly referred to as tooth eruption. It is a complex process that can be influenced by a number of general factors like genetics, nutrition, preterm birth, socioeconomic factors, hormonal factors, various systemic diseases and some local factors. Timing of tooth eruption depends on the chronologic age.[16]

Premature eruption is described as a tooth that has less root development than its projected root length at eruption, according to the diagnostic criteria proposed by Becker. [17] Generalized premature eruption is seen in patients with hyperthyroidism, hypophosphatasia, cherubism, and cyclic neutropenia. Premature eruption of permanent teeth without any systemic condition has also been reported. Early eruption of permanent teeth could be due to premature loss of primary teeth if the loss occurs within 1 year before the eruption.[18]

Prevalence

Nagihan Koc et al (2021) [19] conducted a retrospective study. They selected a sample of 1715 patients aged 5 to 11 years. Panoramic radiographs were used to assess premature eruption and agenesis of premolars. Developmental stage of erupted premolars was assessed using Demirjian's method and selecting prematurely erupted premolars on the basis of clinical eruption with a root length less than half of their final expected root lengths. At the result of the study 115 [6.7%] of 1715 patients, had at least one premolar agenesis, with mandibular second premolars being the most absent. A total of 85 [5.0%] patients had at least one prematurely erupted premolar, most affected by maxillary first premolars.

Etiology

Stephan Christian Möhlhenrich et al (2023) [20] conducted a study to determine the possible relationship between the eruption of primary and permanent teeth and neonatal factors in German children according to gender. A questionnaire was used to gather data on the gender, birth weight (g), height (cm), time of birth (week of pregnancy) and age of first primary and first permanent teeth eruption (months/years) of 405 children (230 girls and 175 boys). For males, there was no association between primary teeth eruption and neonatal characteristics (birth weight, height, and time of delivery). For females, however, there was little association between the eruption of the first primary teeth and height and weight at birth. For either gender, there were no associations between neonatal characteristics and the emergence of the first permanent tooth. The initial primary and first permanent tooth eruptions were shown to be moderately correlated.

Gomes PN et al (2023) [21] did a case-control study to assess whether microcephaly is a risk factor for alterations in the chronology and sequence of tooth eruption and for developmental defects of enamel. 81 children aged 30-36 months, including 40 normoreactive children and 41 with microcephaly, were submitted to oral clinical examination to determine the frequency of alterations in the chronology and sequence of tooth eruption and developmental enamel defects. They concluded that microcephaly was significantly associated with delayed tooth eruption, modifications in the sequence of tooth eruption, and defects in dental enamel.

Hirst Let al (2021) [22] reported a case of a patient with a rare disorder called WDSTS, born at term with feeding difficulties, diagnosed with facial features like telecanthus, flared eyebrows, and palpebral fissures. Her parents were concerned about autistic spectrum features and sensory issues. Testing for the Cornelia de Lange syndrome panel revealed a heterozygous pathogenic variant in the KMT2A gene, confirming the diagnosis of WDSTS. At age 6 years and 9 months, an orthodontic assessment was carried out with an orthopantomogram (OPG). This revealed that all her primary teeth had erupted by eight months and most of the primary teeth had exfoliated between the ages of 24-36 months. The literature describes several oral and dental anomalies in patients with WDSTS, with premature eruption of primary and permanent teeth being commonly cited.

Jha et al (2020) [23] reported a case of premature eruption of premolar in a 7 year old child to the Department of Pedodontics and Preventive Dentistry, Dr. R Ahmed Dental College and Hospital with the chief complain of a male reporting pain in his lower right posterior tooth. Examination revealed decayed 85 and erupted 44. IOPA X-ray showed retained roots and inflammation. Crown formation was almost complete, but root formation had not yet started. 44 had fully erupted without root formation. The patient had a history of intraoral swelling and pus discharge. Rootless teeth are common in cases of dentin dysplasia and localized odontodysplasia, characterized by pulpal obliteration, eruption, radiolucencies, and early exfoliation. In this case, enamel and dentin were healthy, possibly due to decayed primary tooth. The erupting premolars in these cases were mobile. According to Mulia et al., the eruption rate of primary teeth is influenced by the pace of root resorption, but not the formation of permanent teeth.[9] Extensive alveolar bone loss brought on by persistent inflammation emanating from the primary teeth accelerates eruption. This disorder is characterized by an early eruption of the tooth without the formation of a root.

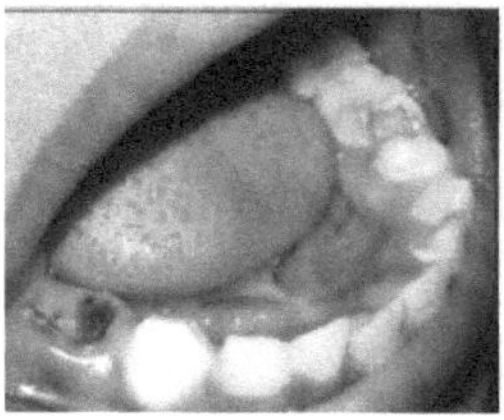

Figure 1 Intraoral picture showing fully erupted first premolar

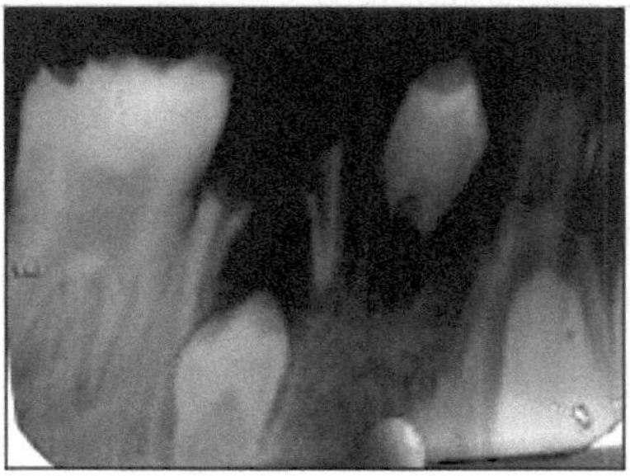

Figure 2 IOPAR showing rootless first premolar

Garmash O (2019) [24] studied the effect of body overweight at birth (fetal macrosomia) on the processes of tooth eruption and tooth growth during the first year of life in children in the Kharkiv City (Ukraine) population. Medical records of babies born from 1977 to 2013 were analyzed. The Kharkiv City database included the medical records of children born with fetal macrosomia, categorized by gender and development coefficient, as well as comparison groups with normal weight and height for the period. According to the study's findings, children with macrosomia had slower deciduous tooth growth rates and more variations in the timing of tooth eruptions than what was typical for the area.

I Gozes et al (2017) [25] conducted a study to determine premature primary tooth eruption in cognitive/motor-delayed ADNP-mutated children. Activity-dependent neuroprotective protein (ADNP) is a frequently mutated ASD gene, protecting nerve cells against electrical blockade. RNA sequencing and gene array analysis reveal dysregulation of bone/nervous system-controlling genes, including BMP1 and BMP4. AKAP6, a major gene regulated by ADNP, links cognition and bone maintenance. This discovery can provide early diagnosis and treatment plans.

Carolina Un Lam et al (2016) [26] did a longitudinal study aiming to influence the metabolic-linked early life factors on the eruption timing of the first primary tooth. Participants were recruited (n = 1033) through the GUSTO (Growing Up in Singapore Towards healthy Outcomes) birth cohort (n = 1237). Oral examinations were performed at 3-month intervals from 6 to 18 months of age. Overall mean eruption age of the first primary tooth was 8.5 (SD 2.6) months. Infant weight gain from birth to 3 months, ethnicity and maternal childbearing age were significant determinants of first tooth eruption timing. The study showed that early life influences can affect primary tooth development, possibly via metabolic pathways.

Chapter-2

DELAYED ERUPTION

Delayed tooth eruption (DTE) is the emergence of a tooth into the oral cavity at a time that deviates significantly from norms established for different races, ethnicities, and sexes.[27] Delayed eruption is defined as a tooth that deviates from the average eruption time by >2 standard deviations .[28] Delayed Tooth Eruption (DTE) is characterized by a variety of terms, but they all refer to the two main factors that affect this phenomenon: (1) biological eruption, which is measured by the development of roots, and (2) expected tooth eruption time (chronologic age), as determined by population studies. [29-31]

When a primary tooth is over-retained past the established period of its normal exfoliation time, it remains in the child's oral cavity and frequently causes a delay in the permanent successor tooth, a condition known as persistent primary tooth (PPT), which is a common clinical condition in children and teenagers. [32,33]

The delayed eruption has been linked to a variety of local variables, including congenitally absent teeth, supernumerary teeth, and malformations. In addition, dilatation, trauma, loss of space, early extraction or loss of primary teeth, and retained primary teeth are common reasons. [34]

The genetic aetiology of primary failure of eruption, an uncommon disorder marked by inadequate tooth eruption even in cases when there is a clear eruption pathway, has been examined by research organizations. It was discovered that 51 different variations of the PTH1R (parathyroid hormone 1 receptor) gene were the primary cause of the eruption failure.[2] According to recent studies there may be a genetic component to the genesis of milder forms of tooth eruption alterations, such as delayed tooth eruption with or without PPT. This common condition may be linked to gene variants (SNPs) in genes such as Matrix metalloproteases 8 (MMP8) [34] and the receptor activator of NF-κB ligand (RANKL).[35]

However, the normal timing and sequence of tooth eruption can be disturbed in people with metabolic bone disorders (MBDs), which frequently results in dental anomalies such as failure of tooth eruption (FTE), delayed tooth eruption (DTE), or premature eruption.[36]

Prevalence

Hummel B et al (2023) [37] conducted this study to utilize panoramic radiographs to determine the prevalence of dental anomalies and developmental disturbances in a heterogenous adolescent orthodontic patient population seeking care at a North American orthodontic residency program. A total of 1042 panoramic radiographs of 457 male and 585 female orthodontic patients aged 10 to 18 years were evaluated. The most common overall finding was agenesis (12.00%), followed by deviations in eruption path (9.12%), delayed eruption (7.39%), and impaction (7.29%). There was no difference in the prevalence of having any anomalous finding or the prevalence of any specific category of anomalies based on the sex or Angle classification of the patients.

Etiology

Del Rio Cantero N (2024) [38] conducted a longitudinal cohort study to determine whether patients with Osteogenesis Imperfecta treated with pamidronate and/or zoledronic acid have a delayed eruption age compared to a control group of healthy children. In their study comparing the age at which the first stage of mixed dentition erupted in a group of 37 Osteogenesis Imperfecta children who were all receiving intravenous bisphosphonates to 89 healthy children, the Pearson correlation test was used to determine the association between the chronology of tooth eruption and the type of medication (zoledronic acid or palidronate) given to the study group. It also established the relationship between the cumulative dose received and tooth eruption. In conclusion, compared to a comparison group of youngsters in good health, patients with OI had a delayed eruption of the first stage mixed dentition. The cumulative dosage of bisphosphonates and the use of zoledronic acid are directly linked to this delayed eruption.

Ji L et al (2024) [39] carried out a study to explore the regulatory effect of RUNX2 mutation on dental follicle cells (DFCs) senescence and clarify the underlying mechanism with aim to explore the basis for a novel mechanism of delayed permanent tooth eruption in cleidocranial dysplasia (CCD) patients. Dental follicles were collected from a cleidocranial dysplasia patient and healthy controls. Senescence-associated β-galactosidase (SA-β-gal) staining, Ki67 staining, cell cycle assays, and senescence-related gene and protein expression assays were performed to assess dental follicle cells senescence. Western blotting was performed to detect the activation of mitogen-activated protein kinase (MAPK) signalling pathways, and the molecular mechanism underlying RUNX2 regulating in dental follicle cells senescence was explored. Consequently, the RUNX2 mutation in cleidocranial dysplasia patients downregulated the expression of senescence-associated genes and proteins, encouraged proliferation, and prevented the cellular senescence of DFCs. Additionally, it inhibited the activation of the ERK signalling pathway. It concluded that the ERK signalling pathway caused by the RUNX2 mutation postponed the senescence of dental follicle cells, which could be the cause of cleidocranial dysplasia patients delayed permanent tooth eruption.

Vaz FFS et al (2023) [40] carried out a study to investigate the impact of severity of microcephaly caused by the Zika virus (MCZ) on tooth eruption and orofacial structures of children. The study included 27 children diagnosed with MCZ. The data was collected in June 2018 through a questionnaire answered by the legal guardians, followed by a clinical examination of the children. A study of 20 children found that 35.0% had severe microcephaly, 30.0% had altered tooth eruption sequence, and 50.0% had delayed eruption. Orofacial changes were most common, but severity did not affect tooth eruption.

The study showed that a failure of delayed tooth eruption is commonly attributed to the presence of a supernumerary tooth.

Seehra J et al (2023) [41] did a systematic review aimed at assessing the percentage of impacted maxillary incisors that successfully erupt after surgical removal of supernumerary teeth with or without other interventions. Systematic literature searches without restrictions were undertaken in 8 databases for studies reporting any intervention aimed at facilitating incisor eruption, including surgical removal of the supernumerary alone or in conjunction with additional interventions published up to September 2022. According to a survey of 15 trials with 1058 individuals, the eruption prevalence was much higher when a supernumerary tooth was removed along with space creation or orthodontic traction (82.4% and 96.9%, respectively) than when an associated supernumerary tooth was removed alone. In the deciduous dentition, the removal of the obstruction in a conical position at the level of the gingival third and with inadequate root growth increased the chances of a successful eruption. Better eruption odds were linked to delaying tooth extraction for 12 months after the eruption period and waiting more than 6 months for spontaneous eruption following the removal of an obstruction.

Kuchler EC et al (2022) [14] conducted a study to evaluate Single Nucleotide Polymorphisms in *COX2*. It is associated with Persistent Primary Tooth and Delayed Permanent Tooth Eruption. Orthodontic treatment children's permanent successor's Nolla stage was assessed using orthopantomographs, with primary tooth retained in Nolla stage 8 and below alveolar crypt, Nolla stage 9, Nolla stage 10. The study involved 100 children, 51 of whom had at least one PPT, and 49 were controls, using saliva samples for DNA extraction and real-time PCR of two SNPs. There were between one and eight teeth that remained in the oral cavity. The co-dominant model linked SNP rs5275 to PPT, with individuals with two T alleles three times more likely to present with PPT than those with at least one C allele. In summary, single nucleotide variations in the COX2 gene was linked to persistent primary teeth and may delay the emergence of permanent teeth.

Bawazir OA et al (2021) [42] reported a case of a 10-year-old child who experienced a delayed tooth eruption after a compound odontoma was surgically removed too late. Odontomas are the most common odontogenic tumors which are usually asymptomatic and discovered during routine radiographic examinations or during an assessment of delayed tooth eruption. Odontomas are classified into compound or complex based on the microscopic structure of dental tissues. A 10-year-old boy's instance with compound odontomas that stopped the permanent mandibular lateral incisor from erupting. The mandibular primary lateral incisors were extracted, and the compound odontomas were surgically removed. At the age of 13, following three years of observation, the permanent lateral incisor burst and came close to the occlusal plane. They came to the conclusion that a delayed eruption of the impacted teeth was caused by the late surgical excision of odontomas.

D' souza VD et al (2021) [43] reported a case of non- syndromic delayed eruption of multiple teeth. A 16-year-old girl with non-syndromic delayed eruption of multiple teeth complained of incorrect tooth positioning for ten years. Her parents complained of tooth crowding. The patient had modest build, diet, no skeletal or physical abnormalities, and no mental retardation.

Mandibular and maxillary deciduous molars were immobile and retained. The patient was referred to a doctor whose supervision included thyroid function tests, in order to rule out any related hormonal abnormalities. The patient was diagnosed with non-syndromic delayed eruption based on the clinical examination and history, due to ankylosed deciduous teeth and congenitally absent permanent teeth. Genetic disease was ruled out, but eruption pattern may be altered by poorly characterized endocrine disease or subclinical hormonal malfunction.

Arid J et al (2019) [35] carried out a study to determine if genetic polymorphisms for RANK/RANKL/OPG are associated with delayed tooth emergence. Saliva samples from 160 children, ages 6 to 13, were examined to see whether genetic variants for RANK/RANKL/OPG could be linked to delayed tooth emergence. Periapical tissue from 15 children with persistent primary teeth and 15 control participants was gathered for qPCR analysis in order to determine whether there is a relationship between the gene expression of RANK/RANKL/OPG in children with delayed tooth emergence and persistent primary teeth. At least one permanent tooth had delayed emergence in 56 children (35%) who had delayed tooth emergence. The genetic polymorphisms rs17099443 and rs3765620 in MMP8, and rs478927 and rs2252070 in MMP13 were genotyped. As a results the polymorphism rs17099443 in MMP8 was associated with delayed tooth eruption in the genotype distribution (P = .05).

Lopes CMI et al (2018) [44] conducted a study to evaluate the prevalence and severity of developmental defects of enamel (DDE) and delayed tooth eruption in children with sickle cell anaemia. The sample comprised 56 male and female children with sickle cell anaemia aged 6 to 12 years and treated at the Hematology and Hemotherapy Center of Pernambuco, Brazil.

The data was collected according to the WHO criteria for DDE and tooth eruption. As a result, the delay increased with age and was detected in 11.8% of children aged 6 to 8 years, in 20.0% of those aged 8 to 10 years and in 54.2% of those aged 10 to 12 years. Prevalence of Delayed tooth eruption was higher in males (36.7%) and showed a significant association with age. Study concluded that sickle cell anemia, a genetic disease caused by a mutation in the beta-globin gene, can present oral manifestations such as delayed tooth eruption and hypomineralized enamel and dentin.

Alsani Aet al (2018) [45] did a study to discuss a case of an 11-year-old pediatric patient, who was diagnosed with delayed eruption of the permanent maxillary central incisors because of palatally impacted supernumerary teeth. Blocking by excess primary teeth and supernumerary teeth may cause the delayed eruption of permanent teeth. Complications can be avoided with an early diagnosis. The position of the teeth, their developmental stage, and the amount of available space all affect how these situations are managed. Orthodontic and surgical procedures may be used in combination for treatment. The primary retained teeth and supernumerary teeth were surgically extracted in two visits to manage the case and the impacted permanent incisors were then left to erupt naturally. They came to the conclusion that, in the absence of orthodontic treatment, the two permanent incisors naturally erupted following an 18-month follow-up.

Psoter WJ et al (2016) [46] carried out a longitudinal study to prospectively evaluate tooth emergence timing between children positive and negative for HIV in the exposed and unexposed groups, respectively. Children positive for HIV and HIV-negative household peers, aged 2 to 15 years was conducted between 1993 and 1996. Emergence status was determined for the maxillary and the mandibular permanent first molars and the central and lateral incisors. A total of 116 participants (62 HIV positive, 54 HIV negative) completed six examinations over the 36-month study period. Statistical differences in tooth emergence timing were observed for five of the six tooth pairs, with children positive for HIV being less likely to have emergence of the corresponding tooth compared with the children negative for HIV. Age differences for each tooth pair ranged from 0.7 to 1.5 years, with a median emergence age difference of 1.03 years. It concluded that delayed tooth emergence of the permanent dentition was observed in children with HIV.

Carvalho IF et al (2016) [47] conducted a study to investigate possible malformations in the soft, bone and/or dental tissues in patients with congenital Zika Virus (ZIKV) by clinical and x-ray evaluation. The study evaluated 30 children with ZIKV and 30 without ZIKV over 24 months, assessing factors such as sex, age, cleft palates, soft tissue lesions, and eruption delay. The study examined 30 babies, with 60% experiencing eruptions after 9 months. The majority had cleft palate, inadequate lingual posture, micrognathia, tooth changes, and muscle spasms. Delayed eruption was associated with inadequate lingual posture, micrognathia, and tooth changes. Female patients had the most narrow palatine vaults, indicating a high prevalence of ZIKV. To draw conclusions the first deciduous tooth's delayed emergence, poor lingual posture, and short labial and lingual frenum's were more common in children with ZIKV.

Chapter-3

Syndromes Associated with Early and Delayed Eruption in Children

Abnormal tooth eruption is linked to a variety of hereditary disorders and systemic syndromes, most of which are caused by harmful gene mutations. Genetic mutations that interfere with dental follicle cells and prevent appropriate tooth eruption cause the following problems among these conditions: Dentin dysplasia brought on by mutations in the VPS4B gene; mucopolysaccharidosis type VI due to mutations in the arylsulfatase B gene; enamel renal syndrome due to mutations in the FAM20A gene and cleidocranial dysplasia linked to mutations in the Runt-related gene 2 gene. Additionally, tooth eruption failure is associated with multiple calcific hyperplastic dental follicles and regional odontodysplasia, but these conditions are unrelated to gene alterations. [48]

Many syndromes have been identified that involve failure of eruption, including cleidocranial dysplasia, Gardner syndrome, osteoglophonic dwarfism, regional odontodysplasia , oculodental syndrome, Rutherfurd type, Nance–Horan syndrome, cherubism, Albers-Schönberg osteopetrosis, McCune–Albright syndrome, hypodontia–dysplasia of nails syndrome, osteopetrosis, mucopolysaccharidosis, MPS I-H, MPS II, MPS VI , GAPO syndrome, Gorlin–Goltz syndrome, McCune–Albright syndrome, osteopetrosis, osteogenesis imperfecta, progeria, sclerosteosis, and hypophosphatemic rickets among others.[2]

A group of diseases known as MBDs impacts bone mass, bone metabolism, and bone quality. Bone mass, structure, and microarchitecture abnormalities caused by these disorders impair bone strength and raise the risk of fractures. As a result, these disorders are linked to an increased risk of severe consequences. These conditions encompass a number of disorders, including cleidocranial dysplasia, Apert syndrome, Gardner syndrome, and amelogenesis imperfecta, that have been demonstrated to result in delayed tooth eruption or even failure of tooth eruption. [49]

Amelogenesis Imperfecta (AI) is the term for hereditary enamel abnormalities that present with a range of genetic patterns and symptoms. Autosomal dominant, autosomal recessive, X-linked recessive, or spontaneous de novo mutation can be the cause of it. Amelogenesis Imperfecta can occur alongside delayed tooth eruption in addition to enamel abnormalities.[50] According to a study by W. Kim Scow, oral eruptive issues, such as follicular cysts and dental impaction, are more common in Amelogenesis Imperfecta and may even result in non-eruption.[51]

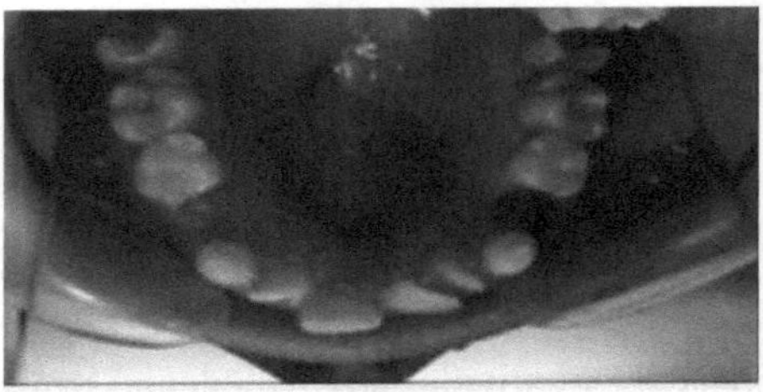

Figure 3 Intraoral view showing the presence of multiple retained deciduous teeth, non-eruption of permanent successors, along with retained root

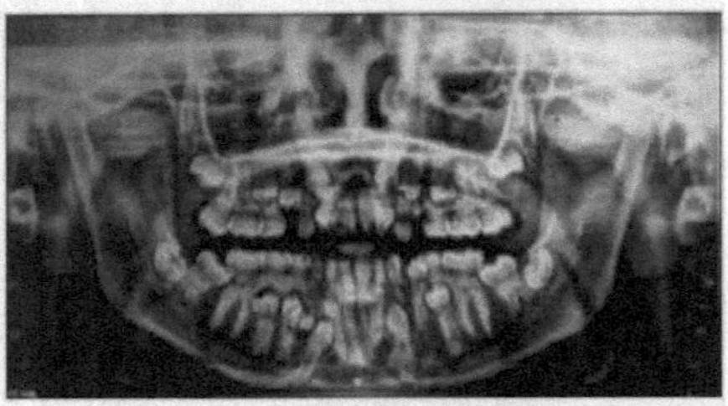

Figure 4 Orthopantomogram of the patient revealed the presence of

multiple impacted and unerupted teeth in both maxillary and mandibular dentition along with failure of root completion

Apert syndrome (Acrocephalosyndactyly type I) is a rare genetic craniosynostosis disorder caused by mutations in the FGFR2 gene. Premature fusion of the cranial sutures, undeveloped midface, and syndactyly of the hands and feet are characteristics that affect TE. [52] Tooth eruption usually occurs 0.96 years later, with a range of 0.5 to 2.9 years. [53,54] The teeth may have crowded and moved within the alveolar bone, causing the delayed eruption. An additional consideration is a primary TE impairment linked to the "mesenchymal disorder" another feature of Apert syndrome.[55]

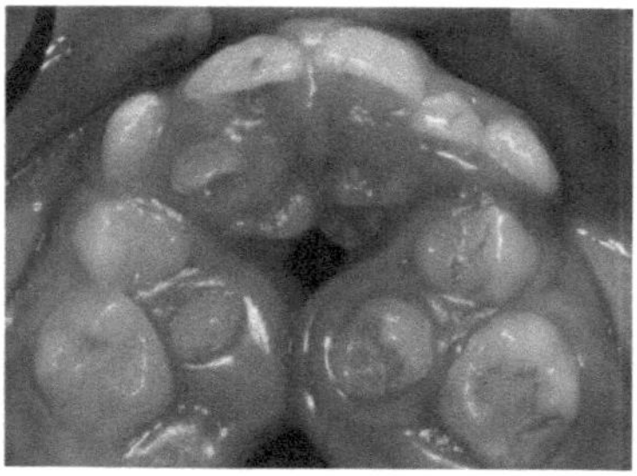

Figure 5. A 12.1-year-old boy with Apert syndrome presented with cleft palate and severe TE disturbances. [53,54]

Carpenter syndrome (acrocephalopolysyndactyly Type II) an autosomal recessive craniosynostosis disorder, is characterized by features such as acromegaly, fusion of the fingers and toes, polydactyly, congenital heart disease, intellectual impairment, hypogonadism, obesity, and umbilical hernia. It may exacerbate TE because of its characteristic craniofacial traits, which include large eyes, a flattened nose, an undeveloped midface, and a protruding forehead. Mutations in the RAB23 gene, which controls the Hedgehog signalling pathway, are the cause. The proliferation and differentiation of dental tissues are impacted by this route, which is important for tooth development.[56] Due to faulty signalling pathways, the disease frequently presents as hypodontia, DTE, a narrow high palate, and the persistence of primary teeth. [57,58]

Cherubism an uncommon, autosomal dominant, inherited, non-neoplastic condition, develop fibrous connective tissue in jaw bones, resulting in bilateral, painless, symmetrical jaw expansion that resembles Renaissance cherubs. It primarily affects the development of bones and teeth, leading to dental anomalies including root resorption, delayed tooth eruption, failure in tooth eruption, and early exfoliation of primary teeth. [59]

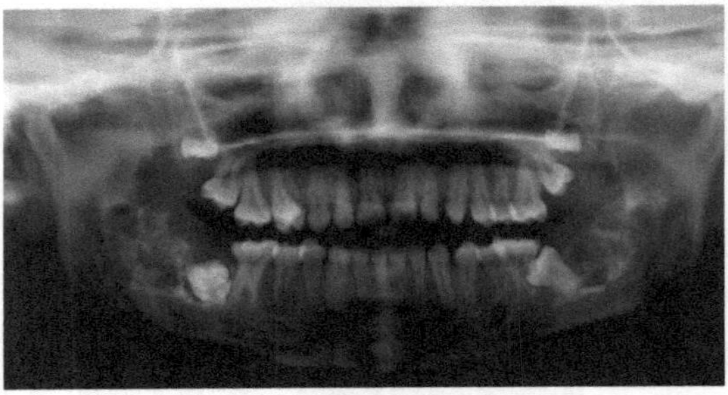

Figure 6. Panoramic radiograph with multilocular irregular radiolucency in the rami sparing the condyle and coronoid, with numerous dental abnormalities: impacted second molars, taurodont first molars, dilacerated 12 and 22, talon cusps in 11 and 21, dens invaginatus in 24, root resorption in 25 and 45 with periapical rarefaction, and a complex odontome lingual to 47. [60]

Cleidocranial dysostosis is an uncommon autosomal dominant genetic condition that is either created de novo or results from mutations in the RUNX2 gene. It is distinguished by small stature, open sutures and fontanelles, aberrant clavicles, and other skeletal abnormalities. A high, narrow palate, orofacial clefts, protracted primary teeth, delayed tooth eruption affecting teeth during their developing phases, and supernumerary teeth (up to 30 teeth) are examples of oral symptoms. [61,62]

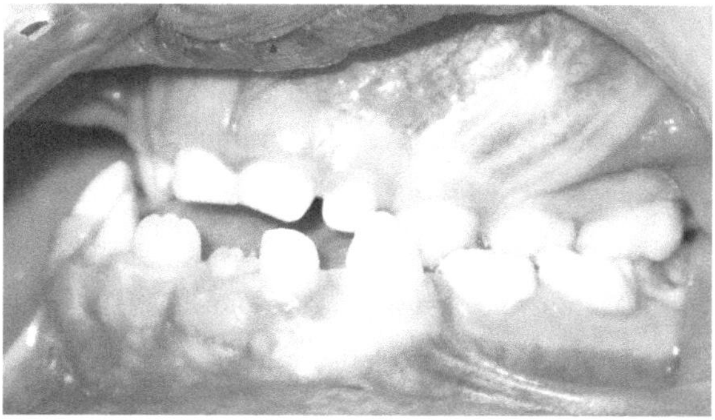

Figure 7 - Intraoral photographs of CCD patient, pre-treatment, 13-year-old boy showing persistence of primary dentition [63]

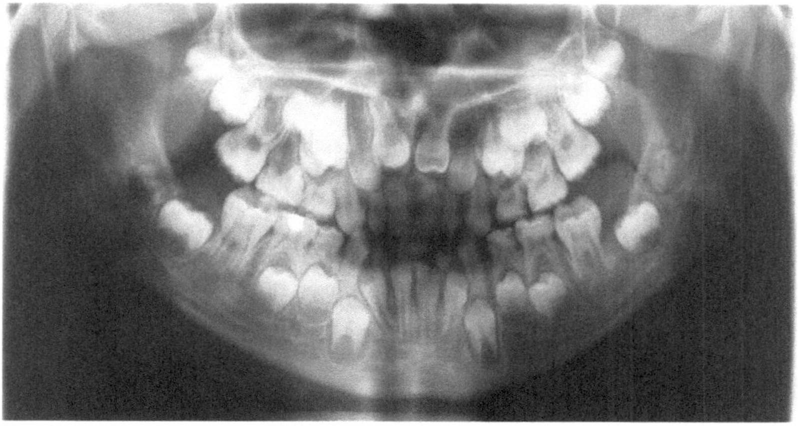

Figure 8. Panoramic radiographs of CCD patient, pre-treatment, 13-year old[63]

Mucopolysaccharidosis Type I-H (MPS I-H), Type II (MPS II), and Type VI (MPS VI) the genetic disorders known as mucopolysaccharidosis types I-H (Hurler), II (Hunter), and VI (Maroteaux–Lamy) are caused by deficiencies in the enzymes α-L-iduronidase, iduronate-2-sulfatase, and N-acetylgalactosamine-4-sulfatase. This leads to the accumulation of glycosaminoglycan, which affects bone metabolism, jaw growth, TE, and potentially fatal vital organ damage. Tooth enamel flaws, DTE, and the suppression of tooth development and eruption are among the orofacial and dental abnormalities that may arise from this buildup of glycosaminoglycans in the gingiva and periodontal tissues. [64-66]

Ectodermal dysplasia is a rare genetic metabolic disorder that affects the growth of ectodermal organs, including the sweat glands, teeth, nails, and hair. Mostly affecting the first stage of tooth development, it frequently results in hypodontia, delayed tooth eruption and irregular tooth shape, along with undeveloped jawbones and a lowered facial height. [67,68]

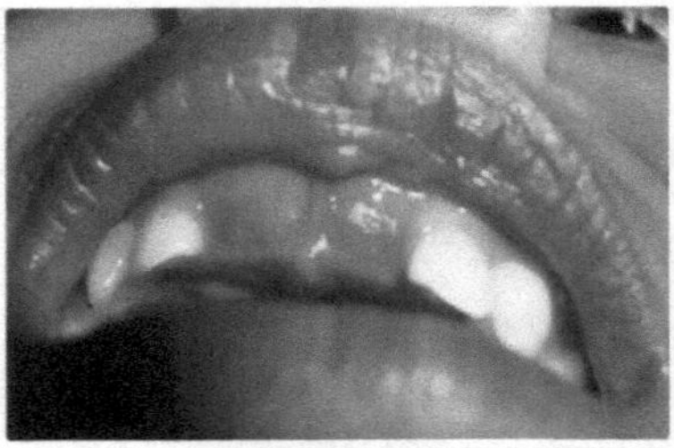

Figure 9: Intraoral examination of the patient revealed unerupted 51, 61, 72, 71, 81 and 82 with overlying thickened fibrous tissue.[69]

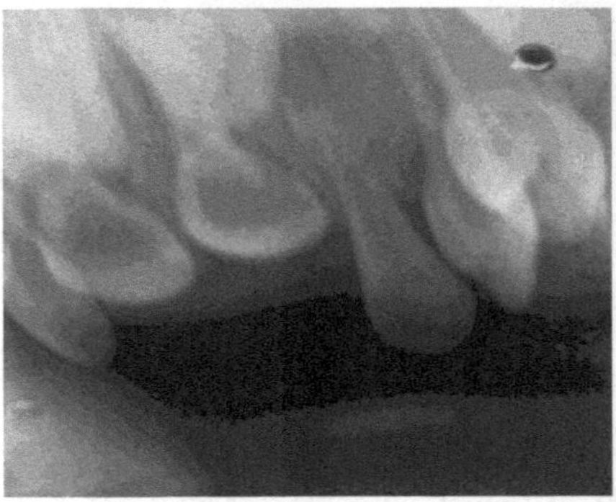

Figure 10: IOPA showing impacted primary maxillary central incisors

GAPO syndrome is a very uncommon autosomal recessive disorder that manifests as ocular atrophy, growth retardation, baldness, and pseudoanodontia. Numerous symptoms, such as micrognathia, delayed bone growth, elevated intracranial pressure, protruding frontal bone, and FTE, may be present in affected individuals. When the early embryonic stages are affected, the teeth do not erupt into the oral cavity even though the tooth buds appear to develop normally within the alveolar bone. [70]

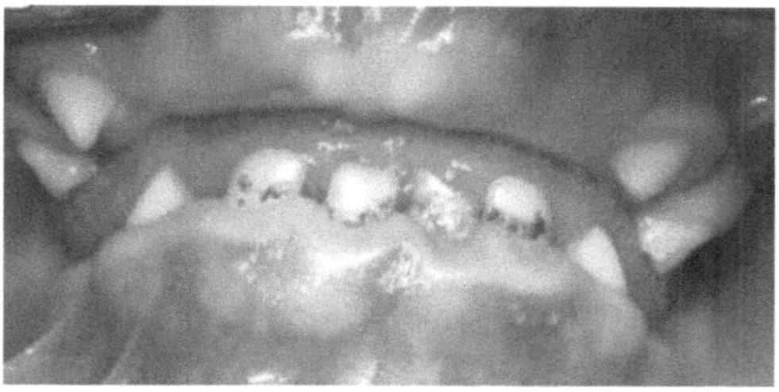

Figure 11: delayed eruption of upper anterior deciduous teeth [71]

Gardner Syndrome is a subtype of autosomal dominant familial adenomatous polyposis (FAP) caused by mutations in the APC (adenomatous polyposis coli) gene. Because of the aberrant growth of both soft and hard tissues in the oral cavity, it significantly affects tooth development and eruption. Tooth agenesis and delayed tooth eruption are among the dental abnormalities that affect 30–75% of individuals. [72]

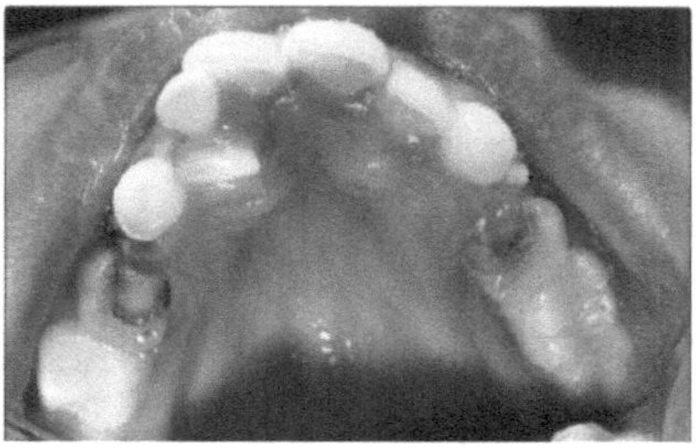

Figure 12: On initial examination at 16 years of age, it was noted that 16 of her permanent teeth had erupted; these teeth displayed normal size, shape, and quality of enamel; 14 of her primary teeth were retained [73]

Gorlin-Goltz syndrome is a rare autosomal dominant disorder caused by mutations in the PTCH1 (protein patched homolog 1) gene. Tumor susceptibility (basal cell carcinomas), odontogenic jaw keratinocysts that affect tooth eruption, delayed tooth eruption, and bone metabolism abnormalities that affect posture and bone health have all been linked to it. [74]

McCune-Albright Syndrome or MAS De novo mutations in the GNAS gene at the postzygotic stage are the cause of McCune-Albright syndrome. Fibrous dysplasia of the craniofacial bones and extra teeth is a common presentation of MAS, which can result in impacted tooth eruption, delayed tooth eruption, and aberrant bone growth. [75-77]

Osteoglophonic dysplasia is a very uncommon autosomal dominant condition that is associated with abnormalities in the fibroblast growth factor receptor 1 gene [*FGFR1*]. Due to the aberrant growth of both hard and soft tissues, it also impacts tooth development and eruption, resulting in oligodontia, delayed tooth eruption, and failure in tooth eruption. [78,79]

Osteopetrosis a rare skeletal illness that can range in severity from asymptomatic to lethal, is characterized by increased bone density brought on by osteoclast malfunction. Ten gene variants are implicated in about 70% of cases. Osteosclerosis, short stature, fractures, injury to the cranial base nerve, and a number of dental anomalies, including tooth agenesis, impaction, FTE, DTE, enamel hypoplasia, or TMJ dysfunction, are frequently the results of this condition. [80,81]

Osteogenesis Imperfecta (OI): Also known as "brittle bone disease," OI is mostly associated with abnormalities in the COL1A1 and COL1A2 genes that impact type 1 collagen, which is essential for bone structure. It is an uncommon autosomal dominant illness.[82] The studies have demonstrated that OI patients receiving bisphosphonates, like zoledronate, present DTE, mainly due to the defective collagen matrix. [83]

Hutchinson-Gilford Syndrome [Progeria] A particular mutation in the

LMNA gene is the primary cause of progeria, an incredibly uncommon autosomal dominant disorder. Cellular division and collagen remodeling are disrupted as a result. Growth retardation, low weight, brachysomia, and disproportionate craniofacial growth, including micrognathia and retrognathia (with mandibular retrognathia being more evident), are early indicators. Teeth development and eruption are delayed as a result. [84-86]

Sclerosteosis is caused by mutations in the SOST gene, which codes for the glycoprotein sclerostin, which prevents bone growth and is the cause of this uncommon autosomal recessive condition. Because of the wider and more dense bones, particularly the cranial bones, DTE patients have bigger jaws and other orofacial anomalies such as forehead and midface hypoplasia and protruding eyes.[87]

Hypophosphatemic rickets is caused by mutation in the PHEX (phosphate-regulating endopeptidase X-linked) gene, a metabolic bone disease that affects individuals of all ages and genders and results in skeletal deformities, growth retardation, and dental problems. DTE, enamel hypoplasia, and tooth abscesses, are some of the symptoms of this illness. [88,89]

Down's syndrome is also known as trisomy 21, trisomy G, and mongolism. An additional copy of chromosome 21 is the source of this autosomal condition, which has an incidence of 1/700. Children with Down syndrome may experience delayed eruption of both primary and permanent teeth. As with the primary dentition, the first eruption in the permanent dentition is delayed, and the same is true for the deciduous dentition. However, the trisomic condition appears to be a determining factor in the delayed eruption in children with Down syndrome. Normal children undergo bone resorption during eruption; children with Down syndrome may experience a slowed rate of this process.[90]

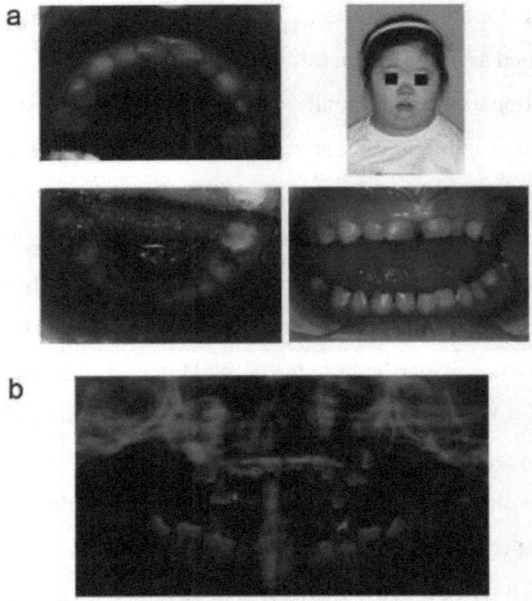

Figure 13. Intraoral view and the facial appearance of the patient at the initial visit demonstrating short neck, short nose and anterior open bite, also the oral status showing a primary dentition with teeth decays and a gingival fistula (a). Panoramic radiograph of the patient at age of 15 years (at initial visit) (b)[90]

Costello Syndrome is a RASopathy that manifests as a variety of developmental, musculoskeletal, dermatological, and cardiac problems. Mutations that activate HRAS are the cause of Costello Syndrome. It is well established that receptor tyrosine kinase (RTK) signalling, which occurs upstream of Ras/mitogen-activated protein kinase [MAPK], is essential for the development of the craniofacial and dental structures. The dental phenotype of Costello Syndrome patients is characterized by malocclusion with anterior open bite and posterior crossbite, gingival hyperplasia, delayed tooth development and eruption, thickening of the alveolar ridge, high palate, and enamel hypo-mineralization. [91]

The non syndromic conditions that affect tooth eruption were identified as: hyperthyroidism, hypothyroidism, hypoparathyroidism, pseudohypoparathyroidism, growth hormone deficiency, and sickle cell anaemia.

Hyperthyroidism in the thyroid hormones triiodothyronine (T3) and thyroxine (T4) cause elevated levels, which can lead to increased metabolic rate, altered hormonal regulation, increased osteoclastic activity, and changes in the dental follicle and periodontal ligament. These changes can impact the intraosseous and extraosseous stages of eruption by speeding up tooth eruption. [92,93]

Hypothyroidism in a thyroid hormone shortage is the hallmark of this condition which can be acquired or congenital. Because of the inadequate development of the mandible and temporomandibular condyles, it might result in dental anomalies as enamel hypoplasia, delayed tooth eruption, micrognathia, and open bite by lowering the metabolic rate and osteoblastic activity. [92,93]

Hypoparathyroidism a rare endocrine condition is characterized by low parathyroid hormone (PTH) levels, which results in hyperphosphatemia and hypocalcemia. Tooth hypocalcemia, tooth hypoplasia, tooth agenesis or impaction, delayed tooth eruption, and short roots are all linked to hypoparathyroidism, depending on the underlying etiology. [94,95]

Pseudohypoparathyroidism's hallmark is the proximal renal tubule's renal epithelial cells' incapacity to react to PTH, which results in excessive hormone release and hypophosphatemia and hypercalcemia.[96] Delayed tooth eruption and other tooth eruption issues are brought on by mutations in the GNAS gene or upstream of the GNAS complex locus. [97,98]

Growth Hormone Deficiency (GHD) Growth and metabolism are impacted by growth hormone (GH), which is produced and released by the anterior pituitary gland.[99] Delayed tooth eruption, which can occur between the ages of 1 and 1.3, is common in children with Growth Hormone Deficiency. This can further delay tooth eruption by affecting bone metabolism and remodelling, which are important processes for tooth eruption. [100,101]

Sickle Cell Anaemia is an inherited hematologic condition, where haemoglobin is changed, resulting in erythrocytes that resemble sickle cells. This causes tissue hypoxia and a shorter cell life. Delayed tooth eruption, pulp calcification, enamel and dentin hypoplasia, bone lesions, oral mucosal pallor, and tongue cell lesions are examples of oral effects. In addition to the general slower growth and development linked to chronic diseases, this delay in tooth eruption may also be caused by regional blood flow abnormalities that impact jaw growth. [102,103]

Dentinogenesis imperfecta (DI) and Dentine Dysplasia are genetic dentin disorders that include two primary types: Based on the clinical classification, Dentinogenesis imperfecta can be further categorized into three subgroups (types I II III), whereas Dentine Dysplasia can be classified into type I (Dentine Dysplasia 1) and type II (Dentine Dysplasia 2). DD1 is a rare autosomal dominant non syndromic disorder in human dentinal diseases, with an estimated incidence of 1/100,000. As a result, delayed tooth eruption is frequently seen in patients with Dentine Dysplasia 1 but is infrequently described as a characteristic of Dentine Dysplasia 2.[104]

Summary

The disturbances in eruption of teeth in children, primary or permanent, and early or delayed, can have a great impact on the child's psychological health. Anxiety of the parents can be understood when the ridges have been edentulous for too long in cases of delayed eruption. Sometimes parents or the primary caregiver might not be aware of what caused the delay in eruption. Rarest of the rare syndromes have been established in literature to hinder the normal eruption process.

While early eruption might not raise alarm for an association with syndromic or genetic conditions like ADND genetic mutation and genes controlling bone regulation namely BMP1 and BMP4. Apart from these, the factors like malnutrition, infant weight and environmental pollutants like dibenzofurans are quite commonly overlooked. (7,25)

Different syndromic conditions alter the timing and course of eruption of both primary and permanent teeth. Among those which are commonly associated with premature and delayed tooth eruption are amelogenesis imperfecta, Apert syndrome, Carpenter syndrome, Cherubism, Cleidocranial dysostosis, Mucopolysaccharidosis, Ectodermal dysplasia, GAPO syndrome, Gardner syndrome, Gorlin-Goltz syndrome, Osteoglophonic dysplasia, Down's syndrome, thyroid disorders and disorders of parathyroid and growth hormone. (50-74,78,79,90,92-101)

Presence of supernumerary teeth and compound odontomas in the oral cavity require surgical intervention as a mode of treatment to facilitate the eruption of teeth. (41,42)

The use of panoramic radiographs/CBCT can help in assessing the status of the unerupted teeth and formulating an appropriate treatment plan. (15,21)

Sound knowledge of the syndromes associated can not only help prepare a definitive diagnosis about the eruption status of the teeth, but also the eruption failure can be traced back retrospectively to find the associated cause and render appropriate treatment.

While most disturbances resolve with time, it is important for parents and caregivers to monitor the child's dental development and seek guidance from a Pediatric dentist if any concern arises. Early intervention and regular dental checkup can help ensure healthy dental growth, prevent complications and promote overall oral health as the child matures.

REFERENCES

1. Proffit W.R., Frazier-Bowers S.A. Mechanism and control of tooth eruption: Overview and clinical implications. Orthod. Craniofacial Res. 2009;12:59–66.
2. Hanisch M., Hanisch L., Kleinheinz J., Jung S. Primary failure of eruption (PFE): A systematic review. Head Face Med. 2018;14:5.
3. Choukroune C. Tooth eruption disorders associated with systemic and genetic diseases: clinical guide. Journal of Dentofacial Anomalies and Orthodontics. 2017;20(4):402.
4. Peedikayil FC. Delayed tooth eruption. e-J Dent. 2011 Oct-Dec; 1(4):81–86.
5. Ataluusua S, Kiviranta H, Leppõniemi A, Hølttõ P, Lukinmaa PL, Lope L, et al. Natal and neonatal teeth in relation to environmental toxicants. Pediatr Res. 2002;52:652–5.
6. Massler M, Savara BS. Natal and neonatal teeth: a review of 24 cases reported in the literature. J Pediatr. 1950;36:349–59
7. Merglova V. Nonsyndromic extremely premature eruption of teeth in preterm neonates–a report of three cases and a review of the literature. Case Reports in Perinatal Medicine. 2018 Aug 28;7(2):20180006.
8. Raghoebar, G.M.; Boering, G.; Vissink, A.; Stegenga, B. Eruption disturbances of permanent molars: A review. J. Oral Pathol. Med.1991,20, 159–166.
9. Proffit W.R., Vig K.W. Primary failure of eruption: A possible cause of posterior open-bite. Am. J. Orthod. 1981;80:173–190.
10. Brandt SK, Shapiro SD, Kittle PE. Immature primary molar in the newborn. Pediatr Dent. 1983;5:210–3.
11. Khatib EK, Abouchadi A, Nassih M, Rzin A, Jidal B, Danino A, et al. Natal teeth: apropos of five cases. Rev Stomatol Chir Maxillofac. 2005;106:325–7.
12. Roulias P, Kalantzis N, Doukaki D, Pachiou A, Karamesinis K, Damanakis G, Gizani S, Tsolakis AI. Teeth Eruption Disorders: A Critical Review. Children (Basel). 2022 May 24;9(6):771.
13. Decker E, Stellzig-Eisenhaurer A, Fiebig BS, et al. PTHR1 loss-of-function mutations in familial, nonsyndromic primary failure of tooth eruption. Am J Hum Genet. 2008;83:781–786.

14. Küchler EC, Henklein SD, Proff P, Lepri CP, Perin CP, Paddenberg E, Roskamp L, Baratto-Filho F, de Menezes-Oliveira MAH, Kirschneck C. Single Nucleotide Polymorphisms in *COX2* Is Associated with Persistent Primary Tooth and Delayed Permanent Tooth Eruption. Int J Environ Res Public Health. 2022 Aug
15. Suri L, Gagari E, Vastardis H. Delayed tooth eruption: pathogenesis, diagnosis, and treatment. A literature review. Am J Orthod Dentofacial Orthop. 2004 Oct;126(4):432-45.
16. Massler M, Schour I. Studies in tooth development: Theories of eruption. Am J Orthod Dentofacial Orthop; 27(10):552-576. 1941.
17. Becker A. Orthodontic Treatment of Impacted Teeth. 3rd ed. West Sussex, UK: Wiley-Blackwell; 5, 2012.
18. Posen AL. The effect of premature loss of deciduous molars on premolar eruption. Angle Orthod. 1965;35:249–52.
19. Koc N, Ballikaya E, Cehreli ZC. Prevalence of Premature Eruption and Agenesis of Premolars in Turkish Children: A Retrospective Study. J Clin Pediatr Dent. 2021 Jan 1;45(1):58-62.
20. Möhlhenrich SC, Korkmaz VC, Chhatwani S, Danesh G. General correlation between neonatal factors, primary and permanent tooth eruption and their interrelation in a population in german orthodontic practices. BMC Oral Health. 2023 Jul 1;23(1):437.
21. Gomes PN, Azevedo ID, do Amaral BA, Arrais NMR, Lima KC. Microcephaly as a risk factor for dental alterations: A case-control study. Oral Dis. 2023 Jul;29(5):2265-2271.
22. Hirst L, Evans R. Wiedemann-Steiner syndrome: A case report. Clin Case Rep. 2021 Jan 5;9(3):1158-1162.
23. Singh P, Jha M. Rootless and prematurely erupted tooth: A case report. J Family Med Prim Care. 2020 Mar 26;9(3):1741-1743.
24. Garmash O. Dependence of Deciduous Tooth Eruption Terms and Tooth Growth Rate on the Weight-Height Index at Birth in Macrosomic Children over the First Year of Life. Acta Medica (Hradec Kralove). 2019;62(2):62-68.
25. Gozes I, Van Dijck A, Hacohen-Kleiman G, Grigg I, Karmon G, Giladi E, Eger M, Gabet Y, Pasmanik-Chor M, Cappuyns E, Elpeleg O, Kooy RF, Bedrosian-Sermone S. Premature primary tooth eruption in cognitive/motor-delayed ADNP-mutated children. Transl Psychiatry. 2017 Feb 21;7(2):e1043.

26.Un Lam C, Hsu CS, Yee R, Koh D, Lee YS, Chong MF, Cai M, Kwek K, Saw SM, Godfrey K, Gluckman P, Chong YS. Influence of metabolic-linked early life factors on the eruption timing of the first primary tooth. Clin Oral Investig. 2016 Nov;20(8):1871-1879.
27.Suri L, Gagari E, Vastardis H. Delayed tooth eruption: pathogenesis, diagnosis, and treatment. A literature review. Am J Orthod Dentofacial Orthop. 2004 Oct;126(4):432-45.
28.Massler M. The development of the human dentition. J. Am. Dent. Assoc. 1941;28:1153.
29.Grøn A.M. Prediction of tooth emergence. J. Dent. Res. 1962;41:573–585.
30.Moorrees C.F., Grøn A.M., Lebret L.M., Yen P.K., Fröhlich F.J. Growth studies of the dentition: A review. Am. J. Orthod. 1969;55:600–616.
31.Aktan A.M., Kara I., Sener I., Bereket C., Celik S., Kirtay M., Ciftçi M.E., Arici N. An evaluation of factors associated with retainede primary teeth. Eur. J. Orthod. 2012;34:208–212.
32.Xavier T.A., Madalena I.R., da Silva R.A.B., da Silva L.A.B., Silva M.J.B., De Rossi A., Küchler E.C., Fukada S.Y. Vitamin D deficiency is a risk factor for delayed tooth eruption associated with retained primary tooth. Acta Odontol. Scand. 2021;79:600–605.
33.Tan C., Ekambaram M., Yiu C.K. Prevalence, characteristic features, and complications associated with the occurrence of unerupted permanent incisors. PLoS ONE. 2018;13:e0199501.
34.Evangelista S.S., Arid J., Vasconcelos K.R.F., Cruz G.V., Dutra A.L.T., da Silva L.A.B., Silva R.A.B., Nelson-Filho P., Vieira A.R., Queiroz A.M., et al. Association between genetic polymorphisms in metaloproteinases of the matrix and delayed tooth emergence: A cross-sectional study. J. Adv. Oral Res. 2019;10:91–96.
35.Arid J., Xavier T.A., da Silva R.A.B., de Rossi A., da Silva L.A.B., de Queiroz A.M., Galo R., Antunes L.A.A., Silva M.J.B., Antunes L.S., et al. RANKL is associated with persistent primary teeth and delayed permanent tooth emergence. Int. J. Paediatr. Dent. 2019;29:294–300.
36.Suri L., Gagari E., Vastardis H. Delayed tooth eruption: Pathogenesis, diagnosis, and treatment. A literature review. Am. J. Orthod. Dentofac. Orthop. 2004;126:432–445.5

37.Hummel B, Yu Q, Frazier J, Ballard RW, Johnson JT, Armbruster PC. The prevalence of developmental dental and eruption anomalies assessed using panoramic radiographs: a retrospective study. Gen Dent. 2023 Jan-Feb;71(1):19-23.
38.Del Rio Cantero N, Mourelle Martínez MR, Sagastizabal Cardelús B, De Nova García JM. Influence of zoledronic acid and pamidronate on tooth eruption in children with osteogenesis imperfecta. Bone. 2024 May;182:117069.
39.Ji L, Li J, Liu D, Qiao Y, Zhao W, Liu Y, Zheng S. RUNX2 mutation inhibits the cellular senescence of dental follicle cells via ERK signalling pathway. Oral Dis. 2024 Apr;30(3):1337-1349
40.Vaz FFS, da Silva Sobrinho AR, Athayde FRRS, de Vasconcelos Carvalho M, Sette-de-Souza PH, Ferreira SJ. Might Zika virus-associated microcephaly's severity impact deciduous tooth eruption and orofacial structures? Oral Dis. 2023 Jul;29(5):2277-2282.
41.Seehra J, Mortaja K, Wazwaz F, Papageorgiou SN, Newton JT, Cobourne MT. Interventions to facilitate the successful eruption of impacted maxillary incisor teeth due to the presence of a supernumerary: A systematic review and meta-analysis. Am J Orthod Dentofacial Orthop. 2023 May;163(5):594-608
42.Bawazir OA. Delayed Eruption of Permanent Lower Lateral Incisor in Relation to Compound Odontoma: A Case Report. J Contemp Dent Pract. 2021 Sep 1;22(9):1060-1062.
43.D'souza VD, Rao PK, Kini R. Nonsyndromic delayed eruption of multiple teeth: A rare case report. J Oral Maxillofac Pathol. 2021 Mar;25(Suppl 1):S51-S53.
44.Lopes CMI, Cavalcanti MC, Alves E Luna AC, Marques KMG, Rodrigues MJ, DE Menezes VA. Enamel defects and tooth eruption disturbances in children with sickle cell anemia. Braz Oral Res. 2018 Aug 13;32:e87.
45.Alsani A, Balhaddad AA. Delayed Eruption of Maxillary Central Incisors Associated with the Presence of Supernumerary Teeth: A Case Report with 18 Months Follow-up. J Contemp Dent Pract. 2018 Dec 1;19(12):1434-1436.
46.Psoter WJ, Nelson EM, Psoter KJ, Dearing BA, Katz RV, Catalanotto F. Delayed tooth emergence in children infected with

human immunodeficiency virus. Oral Surg Oral Med Oral Pathol Oral Radiol. 2016 Oct;122(4):442-7.
47. Carvalho IF, Alencar PNB, Carvalho de Andrade MD, Silva PGB, Carvalho EDF, Araújo LS, Cavalcante MPM, Sousa FB. Clinical and x-ray oral evaluation in patients with congenital Zika Virus. J Appl Oral Sci. 2019 May 20;27:e20180276.
48. Chen J, Ying Y, Li H, Sha Z, Lin J, Wu Y, Wu Y, Zhang Y, Chen X, Zhang W. Abnormal dental follicle cells: A crucial determinant in tooth eruption disorders (Review). Mol Med Rep. 2024 Sep;30(3):168.
49. Papadopoulou CI, Sifakakis I, Tournis S. Metabolic Bone Diseases Affecting Tooth Eruption: A Narrative Review. Children (Basel). 2024 Jun 20;11(6):748.
50. Bin Saleh, S.S. Etiology, Classification, and Restorative Management of Amelogenesis Imperfecta Among Children and Young Adults: A Scoping Review. *Cureus* **2023**, *15*, e49968.
51. Ray JG, Dutta S, Sarangi S, Yadav P. Noneruption of teeth in amelogenesis imperfecta: A report of two cases and review. J Oral Maxillofac Pathol. 2022 Apr-Jun;26(2):254-258.
52. Kaloust, S.; Ishii, K.; Vargervik, K. Dental Development in Apert Syndrome. *Cleft Palate Craniofac. J.* **1997**, *34*, 117–121
53. Hohoff, A.; Joos, U.; Meyer, U.; Ehmer, U.; Stamm, T. The spectrum of Apert syndrome: Phenotype, particularities in orthodontic treatment, and characteristics of orthognathic surgery. Head Face Med. **2007**, 3, 10
54. Renier, D.; Lajeunie, E.; Arnaud, E.; Marchac, D. Management of craniosynostoses. Child's Nerv. Syst. **2000**, 16, 645–658.
55. Droubi, L.; Laflouf, M.; Tolibah, Y.A.; Comisi, J.C. Apert Syndrome: Dental Management Considerations and Objectives. *J. Oral Biol. Craniofac. Res.* **2022**, *12*, 370–375.
56. Hosoya, A.; Shalehin, N.; Takebe, H.; Shimo, T.; Irie, K. Sonic Hedgehog Signaling and Tooth Development. *Int. J. Mol. Sci.* **2020**, *21*, 1587
57. Blankenstein, R.; Brook, A.H.; Smith, R.N.; Patrick, D.; Russell, J.M. Oral findings in Carpenter Syndrome. Int. J. Paediatr. Dent. **2001**, 11, 352–360

58.Kadakia, S.; Helman, S.; Healy, N.; Saman, M.; Wood-Smith, D. Carpenter Syndrome: A Review for the Craniofacial Surgeon. J. Craniofac. Surg. **2014**, 25, 1653–1657. [
59.Kannu, P.; Baskin, B.; Bowdin, S. *Cherubism*; University of Washington: Seattle, WA, USA, 2018.
60.Misra SR, Mishra L, Mohanty N, Mohanty S. Cherubism with multiple dental abnormalities: a rare presentation. BMJ Case Rep. 2014 Oct 9;2014:bcr2014206721.

61.Mundlos S. Cleidocranial dysplasia: Clinical and molecular genetics. J. Med. Genet. 1999;36:177–182.

62.Kolokitha O.-E.G., Papadopoulou A.K. Cleidocranial dysplasia: Etiology, clinical characteristics, diagnostic information and treatment approach. Hell. Orthod. Rev. 2008;11:21–33.
63.Kolokitha, OE., Ioannidou, I. A 13-year-old caucasian boy with cleidocranial dysplasia: a case report. BMC Res Notes **6**, 6 (2013).
64.Mohamed S., He Q.Q., Singh A.A., Ferro V. Mucopolysaccharidosis type II (Hunter syndrome): Clinical and biochemical aspects of the disease and approaches to its diagnosis and treatment. Adv. Carbohydr. Chem. Biochem. 2020;77:71–117.

65.Hirst L., Mubeen S., Abou-Ameira G., Chakrapani A. Mucopolysaccharidosis (MPS): Review of the literature and case series of five pediatric dental patients. Clin. Case Rep. 2021;9:1704–1710.

66.Rodrigues Barros C., Ferrao J., Machado M.D.C., Fernandes A., Proenca F. Hurler Syndrome: Orofacial Clinical Findings. Cureus. 2023;15:e33313.

67.Hekmatfar S., Jafari K., Meshki R., Badakhsh S. Dental management of ectodermal dysplasia: Two clinical case reports. J. Dent. Res. Dent. Clin. Dent. Prospect. 2012;6:108–112.

68.Kearns G., Sharma A., Perrott D., Schmidt B., Kaban L., Vargervik K. Placement of endosseous implants in children and adolescents with hereditary ectodermal dysplasia. Oral Surg. Oral Med. Oral Pathol. Oral Radiol. Endodontol. 1999;88:5–10.

69. Yadiki JV, Kategari YB, Chada P, Vallakatla V. Can Milk Teeth be Impacted? Why Not: A Case of Six Impacted Primary Teeth. Int J Clin Pediatr Dent. 2014 Sep-Dec;7(3):220-2.
70. El-Moataz Bellah Ahmed N, Mostafa MI, Abdel-Hamid MS, Mehrez M. Abnormal dental phenotypes in GAPO syndrome: A descriptive study with a new *ANTXR1* variant & insights on teeth eruption. Saudi Dent J. 2024 Sep;36(9):1209-1214.
71. Sandgren G. GAPO syndrome: A new case. Am. J. Med. Genet. 1995;58:87–90.
72. Cardoso I.L., Gazelle A. Gardner Syndrome: Complications/manifestations in the oral cavity and their relationship with oral health. J. Dent. Open Access. 2020;1:1–7.
73. Bhuvaneswarri J, Chandrasekaran SC. Failure of Eruption of Permanent Tooth. Int J Appl Basic Med Res. 2018 Jul-Sep;8(3):196-198.
74. Nilesh K., Tewary S., Zope S., Patel J., Vande A. Dental, dermatological and radiographic findings in a case of Gorlin-Goltz Syndrome: Report and review. Pan Afr. Med. J. 2017;27:96 .
75. Aravinda K., Ratnakar P., Srinivas K. Oral manifestations of McCune-Albright syndrome. Indian J. Endocrinol. Metab. 2013;17:170–173.
76. Akintoye S.O., Boyce A.M., Collins M.T. Dental perspectives in fibrous dysplasia and McCune-Albright syndrome. Oral Surg. Oral Med. Oral Pathol. Oral Radiol. 2013;116:e149–e155.
77. Xavier S.P., Ribeiro M.C., Sicchieri L.G., Brentegani L.G., Lacerda S.A. Clinical, microscopic and imaging findings associated to McCune-Albright syndrome: Report of two cases. Braz. Dent. J. 2008;19:165–170.
78. Roberts T.S., Stephen L., Beighton P. Osteoglophonic dysplasia: Dental and orthodontic implications. Orthod. Craniofac. Res. 2006;9:153–156.
79. Marzin P., Baujat G., Gensburger D., Huber C., Bole C., Panuel M., Finidori G., De la Dure M., Cormier-Daire V. Heterozygous FGFR1 mutation may be responsible for an incomplete form of

osteoglophonic dysplasia, characterized only by radiolucent bone lesions and teeth retentions. Eur. J. Med. Genet. 2020;63:103729.

*80.*Lam D.K., Sándor G.K., Holmes H.I., Carmichael R.P., Clokie C.M. Marble bone disease: A review of osteopetrosis and its oral health implications for dentists. J. Can. Dent. Assoc. 2007;73:839–844.

81.Stark Z., Savarirayan R. Osteopetrosis. Orphanet J. Rare Dis. 2009;4:5.

82.Marom R., Rabenhorst B.M., Morello R. Management of endocrine disease: Osteogenesis imperfecta: An update on clinical features and therapies. Eur. J. Endocrinol. 2020;183:R95–R106.

83.Cantero N.D.R., Martínez M.R.M., Cardelús B.S., García J.M.D.N. Influence of zoledronic acid and pamidronate on tooth eruption in children with osteogenesis imperfecta. Bone. 2024;182:117069.

84.Gordon L.B., Brown W.T., Collins F.S. Hutchinson-Gilford Progeria Syndrome. University of Washington; Seattle, WA, USA: 2019.

85.Pollex R., Hegele R.A. Hutchinson–Gilford progeria syndrome. Clin. Genet. 2004;66:375–381

86.Domingo DL, Trujillo MI, Council SE, Merideth MA, Gordon LB, Wu T, Introne WJ, Gahl WA, Hart TC. Hutchinson-Gilford progeria syndrome: oral and craniofacial phenotypes. Oral Dis. 2009 Apr;15(3):187-95.

87..Stephen L., Hamersma H., Gardner J., Beighton P. Dental and oral manifestations of sclerosteosis. Int. Dent. J. 2001;51:287–290.

88.Rabbani A., Rahmani P., Ziaee V., Ghodoosi S. Dental problems in hypophosphatemic rickets, a cross-sectional study. Iran. J. Pediatr. 2012;22:531.

89.128.Murayama T., Iwatsubo R., Akiyama S., Amano A., Morisaki I. Familial hypophosphatemic vitamin D-resistant rickets: Dental findings and histologic study of teeth. Oral Surg. Oral Med. Oral Pathol. Oral Radiol. Endodontol. 2000;90:310–316.

90. Wang Y, Zhao Y, Ge L. Delayed eruption of permanent teeth in an adolescent with Down's syndrome: A case report. Journal of Medical Cases. 2015 May 20;6(6):277-8.
91. Goodwin AF, Oberoi S, Landan M, Charles C, Massie JC, Fairley C, Rauen KA, Klein OD. Craniofacial and dental development in Costello syndrome. Am J Med Genet A. 2014 Jun;164A(6):1425-30.
92. Vitalle M.S.d.S., Weiler R.M.E., Niskier S.R., Braga J.A.P. Delayed tooth eruption in an adolescent with hypothyroidism. Rev. Paul. Pediatr. 2012;30:613–616.
93. Little J.W. Thyroid disorders. Part I: Hyperthyroidism. Oral Surg. Oral Med. Oral Pathol. Oral Radiol. Endodontol. 2006;101:276–284.
94. Shimada A., Shibata T., Komatsu K. Relationship between the tooth eruption and regional blood flow in angiotensin II-induced hypertensive rats. Arch. Oral Biol. 2004;49:427–433.
95. Carlos L., Jimenez Soriano Y., Sarrion Perez M.G. Dental management of patients with endocrine disorders. J. Clin. Exp. Dent. 2010;2:e196–e203.
96. Pinto A., Glick M. Management of patients with thyroid disease: Oral health considerations. J. Am. Dent. Assoc. 2002;133:849–858.
97. Kamarthi N., Venkatraman S., Patil P.B. Dental findings in the diagnosis of idiopathic hypoparathyroidism. Ann. Saudi Med. 2013;33:411–413.
98. Reis M.T.A., Matias D.T., de Faria M.E.J., Martin R.M. Failure of tooth eruption and brachydactyly in pseudohypoparathyroidism are not related to plasma parathyroid hormone-related protein levels. Bone. 2016;85:138–141.
99. Hejlesen J., Underbjerg L., Gjørup H., Bloch-Zupan A., Sikjaer T. Dental findings in patients with non-surgical hypoparathyroidism and pseudohypoparathyroidism: A systematic review. Front. Physiol. 2018;9:376009.
100. Atreja G., Atreja S.H., Jain N., Sukhija U. Oral manifestations in growth hormone disorders. Indian J. Endocrinol. Metab. 2012;16:381–383.

101. Torlińska-Walkowiak N., Majewska K.A., Kędzia A., Opydo-Szymaczek J. Clinical Implications of Growth Hormone Deficiency for Oral Health in Children: A Systematic Review. J. Clin. Med. 2021;10:3733.

102. Girgis S., Cheng L., Tsitsikas D., Sproat C. Orofacial manifestations of sickle cell disease: Implications for dental clinicians. Br. Dent. J. 2021;230:143–147.

103. Kelleher M., Bishop K., Briggs P. Oral complications associated with sickle cell anemia: A review and case report. Oral Surg. Oral Med. Oral Pathol. Oral Radiol. Endodontol. 1996;82:225–228.

104. Barron MJ, McDonnell ST, Mackie I, Dixon MJ. Hereditary dentine disorders: dentinogenesis imperfecta and dentine dysplasia. Orphanet J Rare Dis. 2008 Nov 20;3:31.

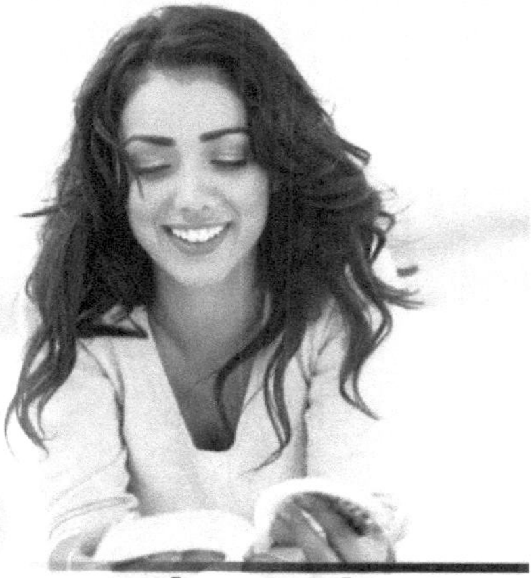

FSC
www.fsc.org
MIX
Papier | Fördert gute Waldnutzung
FSC® C083411

Kolibri 360 GmbH
Ferdinand-Jühlke-Straße 7
99095 Erfurt, Deutschland
produktsicherheit@kolibri360.de

Druck:
CPI Druckdienstleistungen GmbH
im Auftrag der
Kolibri 360 GmbH
Ferdinand-Jühlke-Str. 7
99095 Erfurt